# Eat and Live Healthy

**The Natural Weight Loss Solution**

By: Timothy Campbell

9781635010459

# PUBLISHERS NOTES

## Disclaimer – Speedy Publishing LLC

This publication is intended to provide helpful and informative material. It is not intended to diagnose, treat, cure, or prevent any health problem or condition, nor is intended to replace the advice of a physician. No action should be taken solely on the contents of this book. Always consult your physician or qualified health-care professional on any matters regarding your health and before adopting any suggestions in this book or drawing inferences from it.

The author and publisher specifically disclaim all responsibility for any liability, loss or risk, personal or otherwise, which is incurred as a consequence, directly or indirectly, from the use or application of any contents of this book.

Any and all product names referenced within this book are the trademarks of their respective owners. None of these owners have sponsored, authorized, endorsed, or approved this book.

Always read all information provided by the manufacturers' product labels before using their products. The author and publisher are not responsible for claims made by manufacturers.

*This book was originally printed before 2014. This is an adapted reprint by Speedy Publishing LLC with newly updated content designed to help readers with much more accurate and timely information and data.*

Speedy Publishing LLC

40 E Main Street, Newark, Delaware, 19711

Contact Us: 1-888-248-4521

Website: http://www.speedypublishing.co

REPRINTED Paperback Edition: ISBN: 9781635010459

Manufactured in the United States of America

# DEDICATION

This book is dedicated to everyone who has health issues and challenges.

# TABLE OF CONTENTS

# CHAPTER 1 - LOSING WEIGHT NATURALLY

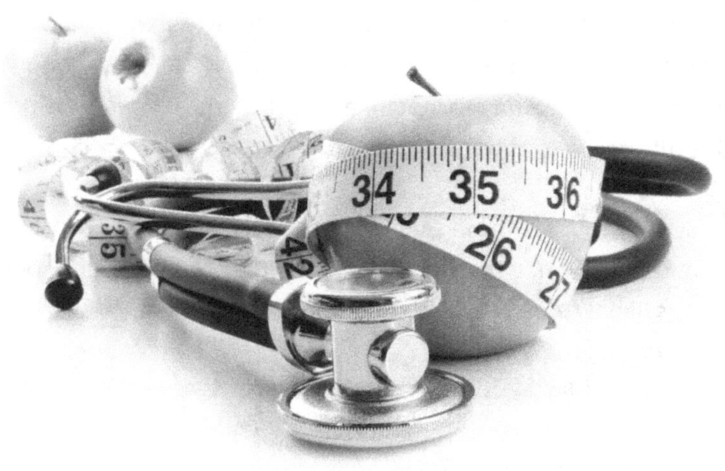

It is a widely recognized and acknowledged fact that the population of most developed Western countries is getting fatter, and we are not talking about a gradual increase here.

The number of people who are seriously overweight or clinically obese is exploding all over the Western world.

Just as an example, the statistics page of the 'Weight-control Information Network' quotes data from the National Health and

Nutrition Examination Survey (NHANES) which indicates that by the end of 2004, around two thirds of adults in the USA were officially overweight, and nearly one third were clinically obese. The situation has already deteriorated significantly since then, so we really do have a global crisis on our hands.

This explosion is placing a very heavy additional burden on the already overworked and under resourced health services in a number of countries.

At the same time, statistics over the past few years would strongly suggest that the trend for citizens of most developed countries to get fatter by the day is not likely to be reversed any time soon without dramatic action.

Consequently, the strain on health services across the world is also going to increase, which in turn means that the inevitable breaking point is likely to be reached soon.

This means that if you are seriously overweight or obese, grabbing your copy of 'Losing weight nature's way' is important, because this represents a significant step forward in a couple of very important ways.

Firstly, it indicates that you or somebody that is close to you – perhaps a family member or other loved one – has a weight problem.

Furthermore, if the individual with the problem is you rather than someone else, this also indicates that you have acknowledged your problem, which is often the first and hardest step.

Secondly, the fact that you are reading this now indicates that you have decided to do something about your weight problem, and that decision represents a very significant shift in your way of thinking and attitude to the shape that you are in.

I don't know many overweight or obese people who are happy with their physical condition, but I do know plenty of people who are seemingly content to put off their decision to start losing weight to another day. Unfortunately for people like this, another day never comes, either because they simply choose to ignore their problem or because their weight problem is a primary factor that helps to kill them off early.

I make no apology for putting it in such blunt, stark terms, because as suggested, people who are significantly overweight or obese represent an increasingly troublesome burden on global society.

The day when health services collapse under the weight of treating people whose problems are generally a result of their own self-indulgence and inability or unwillingness to curb their bad habits is not far away if we don't start reversing the trend towards obesity very soon.

I know that there are hospitals in the UK (which has a National Health Service that is supposed to offer treatment to all, remember) that are already refusing to provide treatment to people who are seriously overweight or obese. I am certain that this is a trend that is likely to become far more common in the years to come, and not only in the UK.

Perhaps you live in a place where you pay for medical attention and treatment, so you might say that this will never happen to you as long as you are willing to pay for your treatment.

Fine, but what happens when your bill doubles or triples because you are seriously overweight or obese?

It's going to happen because the risks involved in undergoing serious medical treatment are significantly higher for overweight or obese people, and you can be sure that if they are not already doing so, the medical authorities will start factoring this into the amount that they charge.

You are reading this, so I take that as a sign that you do not want to be overweight or obese forever.

It is no big secret that after 'make money online' information, the #1 category of information that people are searching for on the internet is weight loss related information.

Consequently, it is also no surprise that there are millions of dollars being spent every day on advertising all sorts of diet plans (of widely varying credibility and effectiveness), weight loss wonder pills and equipment - all of which is supposed to help you lose weight - such as exercise machines, multi-gyms etc.

Some of the diet plans that are advertised are entirely natural but the majority is not. Similarly, most diet pills are not formulated using only natural substances.

There is no shortage of businesses that are advertising their weight loss surgery services, many of them in overseas countries where the cost of medical treatment and attention is considerably less than it is in most Western countries.

While you will read of some almost 'too-good-to-be-true' weight loss surgery success stories, you are far less likely to hear anything about the hundreds of cases where weight loss surgery was ultimately ineffective. It is also a fact that undergoing surgery when you are seriously overweight or obese carries significantly heightened risks, but this again is something that you don't hear about.

Taking chemical-based diet pills or undergoing invasive and thoroughly unpleasant surgery is not natural in any way.

So, now you have a fairly clear idea of some weight loss strategies that could in no way qualify as being natural, let's start to look at the flipside.

**Obese vs. Overweight**

When someone is overweight, their weight exceeds the normal standards for people of their height and age. However, because everyone's weight must include their bones, muscles, fat and water content, it is possible for someone to be overweight without being obese.

For example, a professional athlete or bodybuilder may well be overweight, but because the majority of the 'excess' weight that they are carrying is muscle tissue, they are not obese.

Nevertheless, in the majority of cases, being overweight does equate to carrying too much body fat and often progresses to become clinical obesity.

There are several ways of defining obesity, but the most common is by reference to what is known as 'Body Mass Index' (BMI) which is a mathematical formula that generates a numerical BMI based on an individual's weight in kilograms divided by their height in meters squared. Hence, the mathematical formula for BMI is kg/m2.

The most common way of quantifying whether someone is obese or not is if their BMI is in excess of 30 points on these scales.

**Is It Really Bad as it Appears?**

I would suspect that there are very few people who watch TV or read a newspaper that are not already aware that the problem of obesity is exploding on an international scale.

Consider the following charts taken from the 'U.S. Obesity Trends 1985- 2 0 07' page of the 'Centers for Disease Prevention and Control' (CDC) website.

Although there were a handful of states for which there was no data available, you can see that there was no state in the USA where more than 14% of adults were obese.

Fast forward 10 years, and the picture is looking considerably less encouraging:

Now, there is not a single state where the rate of adult obesity is less than 10%, and there are many who are already in the 15% to 19% adult obesity 'band'.

But if you thought that was bad, take a look at the last available chart from 2007 (from which point, writing this two years further down the line, it is fairly safe to assume that the picture had deteriorated considerably further):

Now, there is only Colorado where there is not more than 20% of the adult population that is clinically obese. And yet, only eight years before that, there wasn't one single state where obesity was already above 20%.

Could anybody need any more proof that obesity is tantamount to an epidemic?

I'm not telling you this try to scare you, because if you are seriously overweight or obese, you already know that you need to do something sooner rather than later. However, just realize that you are not alone in your current predicament, but that you are probably unusual in seeking an answer for your problem.

# Chapter 2- Natural Healthy Lifestyle, a Better You

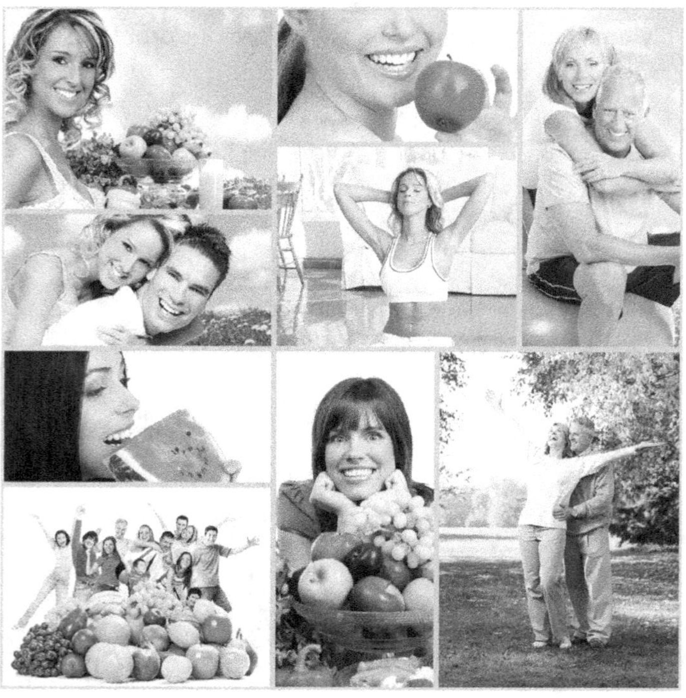

The concept that underpins weight loss or indeed weight gain is a very simple one.

Every human being at every stage of their life needs to take in a certain amount of energy in order to get through the day. This energy comes from the nutrition that we take in, in the form of the food we eat or the liquids we drink, and is generally measured in terms of calories or kilocalories. There is a slight difference between the specific meanings accorded to these two terms, with the latter being favored by professional nutritionists, but for the purposes of this book, I am going to use calories as an all-encompassing unit of food energy.

While every individual is different, you need a certain amount of food energy calories every day to satisfy your own personal energy requirements. These requirements will vary according to the amount of physical work you do, how much exercise you take, the speed at which your body burns the energy you are taking on board (your metabolic rate) and your general lifestyle.

However, at the end of the day, if you take on board the right amount of calories every day, your weight will stay stable and you will in general remain healthy.

If you take in too much energy, you will put weight on, but if you take in too little, you will see the opposite effect and lose weight.

It really is as straightforward as this.

You will see diet plans that recommend that you must cut down on your carbohydrates in order to lose weight, with other diet 'experts' on the opposite side of the fence who swear that the only way to lose weight is to reduce the amount of fats in your diet.

However, no matter what type of food you are eating for energy (which includes both carbohydrates and fats), you are going to keep getting fatter as long as you are taking in more energy than you burning. Thus, you will only lose weight if you are taking in less energy than you need.

That really is it. That is how you lose weight naturally – you ingest less energy than you need every day, and the fat will gradually fall off.

**How much energy do you need?**

Everyone is different. In addition to our physical attributes, every individual has different energy requirements. In addition, there is some evidence that ability to lose or gain weight is to some extent predetermined by your genetic makeup, and there is not a great deal that you can do about changing that.

On top of your genes, there are many external factors that affect how many calories you need, so any standardized 'calorie table' can be nothing other than a very general, broad brush indication of the number of calories that you need.

In order to get a more accurate picture of exactly how many calories you need, you need to factor in many variables, and after considering what these variables are, you will see how you do this.

Firstly, there are the lifestyle factors to take into account, such as the work that you do, the exercise you take and so on.

These are to a large extent taken into account in the underlying calculation on which the previous chart is based. Someone who is working in a sedentary office based occupation is going to need considerably fewer calories every day than someone who is working on a building site, as an example.

In addition to this, however, your present weight and age will also have an influence on the number of calories you need to maintain your current weight levels.

The more weight you are carrying, the more energy you need to get that bulk moving, while as you get older, your energy requirements gradually decrease as you are likely to engage in less physically activity than you did when you were younger.

Gender is also an influential factor, because women generally need fewer calories than men.

Taking all of these variables into account, what you are looking to do is calculate a 'Body Mass Ratio' (BMR) which is not the same as the 'Body Mass Index' that we were considering earlier.

While this book is talking about losing weight, I want to be more specific than this, because I am really talking about losing fat rather than just weight.

As I mentioned earlier, it is possible to be overweight but to have a very low fat to body weight ratio at the same time, because you are carrying a great deal of muscle. In other words, it is possible to be healthy but weigh more than the 'norm'.

There is a common myth that muscle weighs more than fat, but it doesn't. Five pounds of muscle weighs exactly the same as five pounds of fat, but fat is far bulkier than muscle.

Because fat is bulkier, if you are carrying too much fat, you will tend to look 'lumpy' and carrying too much fat brings increased risks to your general health and well being.

So, be clear about this. This book is about losing fat naturally, but if you want to replace that fat with muscle that is fine - because what I am essentially focused on here are your health, well being and fitness.

It's all about shedding fat, getting you as lean, fit and well as possible. That point having been clarified, let's move on.

Part of our natural, basic human makeup means that we tend to store fat. In fact, this is something that has been with us for many thousands of years as it was probably a survival mechanism to get over the times when our ancient forebears were short of food.

Given that it is only in recent times that food has become so abundantly plentiful (at least for those of us who live in the West), we have never really lost the capacity for storing unused energy as body fat.

It is a little like animals that hibernate for the winter. They build up a huge store of unused energy during the summer that is sufficient to keep their inactive body 'ticking over' during the winter months when they are hibernating.

You cannot change, nor can you ignore, thousands of years of evolution. The fact is, modern Western man (and woman) has no real need to store unused energy in the way that our prehistoric forebears did, but you are going to continue doing so despite this.

So, if you are taking on too much energy, you are going to get fat, there is no avoiding this. You therefore need to know an awful lot more about why it happens if you want to tackle your problem entirely naturally.

The first thing that you need to understand about losing weight is that almost everything you eat and drink contains calories. The only exception to this rule in terms of naturally occurring substances is water (more about water later).

Other than that, everything you consume contains calories, and it doesn't really matter a great deal how these calories are taken.

This is one of the reasons why there are so many virulent arguments between those who suggest that in order to lose weight, you need to cut down on carbohydrates and those who on the other hand suggest that fats are the real demon that needs to be banished from your diet, and why they are probably on the wrong track.

There is little quantifiable scientific proof that following one particular eating approach like this is likely to be more effective for losing weight than anything else. While it is not at all difficult to find seemingly qualified people like medical doctors who will tell you that one particular diet regime (e.g. a carbohydrate only diet) is going to help you lose weight more quickly than anything else, it is surely no coincidence that most of these 'objective' observers have some kind of vested interest in the product or proposal that they are supporting.

The fact is, both carbohydrates and fats are processed by the body to produce energy, and so it follows that if you eat too many of either one or the other or even both, you are going to put more weight on.

According to Dr. Kristine Clark (Ph.D., R.D. & FACSM), who is the Director of Sports Nutrition for Penn State University's Athletics Department, one pound of stored fat in the body is equivalent to 3500 calories (which means that every kilo of stored fat is 7700 cal.).

It does not matter a great deal what kind of foodstuffs or drinks are being taken in to accumulate these extra pounds or kilos - for every excess pound of weight you are dragging around, you must take in 3500 calories less than you need to drop that pound.

However, there is one other thing to take into account, which does lend some credence to the people who suggest that taking in energy in 'form A' (e.g. fats) rather than in 'form B' (e.g. carbohydrates) makes you less fat.

This is the fact that our bodies have the ability to process some calories in one way while dealing with others in a completely different manner.

For example, almost despite what we are generally led to believe, our bodies do not necessarily extract all the goodness (vitamins, nutrients etc) or all of the calories from every single item of food we consume.

This happens because your body has its own metabolic rate, a speed at which it processes the food that you take in.

At the same time, while any foodstuff is still within your body, your body will keep extracting as many calories of energy from that food as possible. Consequently, it follows that anyone whose system passes the food through very quickly is going to draw less calories from their food than would someone whose system is more lethargic.

It is probably no great secret that the modern Western diet is far too rich in processed, refined foods and far too light on raw, nutrient packed foodstuffs. We probably all understand that processed foods (burgers, hot dogs, pizzas etc) are likely to make you fatter than raw unprocessed foods, but one of the reasons why this happens is probably not widely understood.

Partially because these foodstuffs are very rich in fats and sugar, our system is simply not very good at processing them. Consequently, they can hang around in your body for two or three days, and while they are still being slowly digested in this way, your body is still leeching every available calorie from them.

Raw foodstuffs on the other hand tend to 'hang around' for only a few hours and therefore, even if they were 'calorie rich' (which most raw foods are not), your body simply does not get the chance to extract those calories.

When you think about it in these terms, it probably makes a great deal of sense. After all, you have spent years listening to people who have told you how good raw and unprocessed foods were for your digestive system. Plus, there have probably been times when the speed at which you have had to visit the bathroom has provided ample testament to the fact that raw food 'keep you going'!

Now you understand why, and you can probably understand why processed or refined foods are likely to help pile the weight on as well. You'll learn more about this concept later.

In contrast, there are other foodstuffs like the essential fatty acids (the Omega-3 and Omega-6 families) that are never likely to add a great deal of fat to your frame no matter how much of them you eat because their primary function is to help with the repair of bodily cells as well as helping to keep many essential metabolic processes functioning correctly.

So, refined foods are likely to add more weight than are natural raw foods even if they have no difference in terms of total calorific value.

You now know what you have to do to start shifting your unwanted flesh – you have to drop around 3500 calories to get rid of one pound of weight or 7700 calories for every kilo.

Here is a final thing to consider before moving on, one very important thing that you must do before embarking on your fat loss program.

It is extremely important that when you initially start your weight loss regime – hopefully immediately after reading this book – you have a final target weight as an objective.

If you do not have a final objective in mind when you start, it is going to be almost impossible for you to ever feel satisfied with the weight that you have lost and the shape you are in.

It can be extremely tempting to just keep losing weight for the sake of it and that is not the way to good health, fitness and general well-being. On the contrary, it is the way to acquiring anorexia, and while I have no doubt that anyone who is seriously overweight or obese might like to believe that they would welcome being anorexic, it is definitely not something you should want.

Without a final target weight in mind, it is far too easy to become obsessed with losing just a pound or two more until one day someone points out to you that you are already way too thin, by which time it is likely that anorexia is already a problem.

I know that you are probably reading these words thinking 'that could never happen to me' but that are what every anorexic person thinks.

So, taking account of your build, bone structure and musculature, try to establish a 'good weight' (note, not an 'ideal' weight – it does not exist) for someone of your build using a weight table such as this or a downloadable, printable chart like this one, and make that your target.

Having done so, stick to that target so that once you get there, you alter your weight loss diet and exercise regime to one that is designed to maintain weight rather than lose it.

Okay, with that note of caution out of the way, let's start to consider what you can do to get rid of those extra pounds.

The answer is really very simple…

You pile on the poundage because you are taking in energy that you are not using.

There are two things that you can do to start shedding the fat pounds, two things that can be done in isolation but which work far better if done together.

One is to increase the amount of calories that you burn every day through a program of sensible exercise.

The second is to reduce the calories that you take in, so that instead of eating more calories than you need every day, you are eating fewer.

As suggested, these could be considered an 'either/or' choice, but I would strongly suggest that you should think about both at the same time, because doing so cannot fail to accelerate the speed at which you will shed the extra pounds.

We will begin by looking at the benefits of exercise.

# Chapter 3- Keep Active

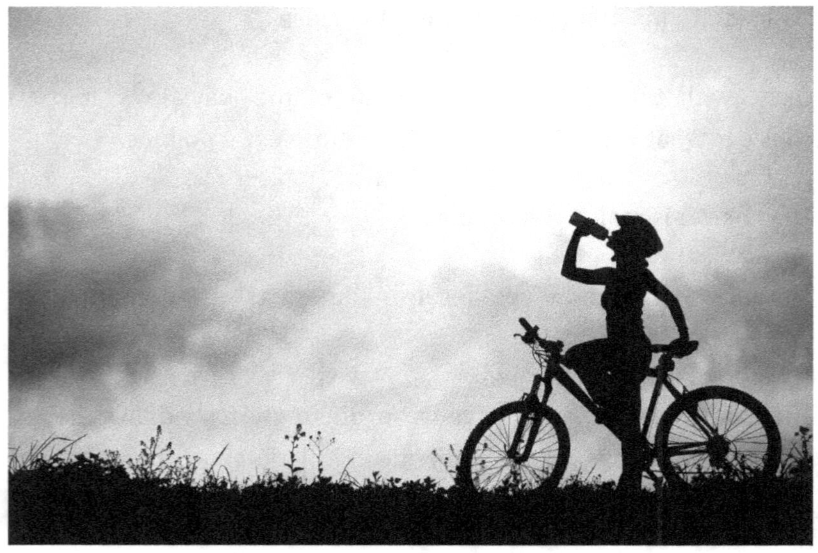

Why exercise helps weight loss in more ways than one

The benefit of exercise is that while you are exercising, you will be burning additional calories over and above those that you have been using previously.

Consequently, exercise will help to get rid of the additional weight you are carrying. If regular exercise and you have become strangers in the recent past, it is time to start getting yourself reacquainted with doing some exercise.

However, it goes much further than actually burning off more calories when you are participating in exercise, because activity helps to speed up your metabolism as well.

In essence, once you start a program of regular exercise, your body might actually burn more calories even when at rest, so that there will be an all-round improvement in the speed at which you are using up the calories. In fact, this improvement can go as far as burning off more calories when you sleep, because although your body is at rest, the 'speed up' effect in your metabolism is a 24/7 thing.

However, it is generally believed that anaerobic exercise is far more effective for burning fat when you are at rest than is aerobic exercise. I will expand on the differences below.

**What kind of exercise is best?**

There is no one answer to the question of what kind of exercise is best, because to a large extent it will depend on what you want to achieve while getting rid of the surplus poundage.

For example, while most overweight people are likely to be primarily interested in getting rid of their surplus fat and not a great deal more, there will be some people who are equally interested in building their musculature.

For anyone that falls into this category, the exercises that you choose to do will be different from those that work best for people who are just trying to shed the extra pounds of fat. As an example, if you are trying to replace fat with muscle, then lifting weights is going to be more appropriate than would be swimming or running, although of course, all three forms of exercise would have significant benefits.

In essence therefore, you need to know what your primary target is before deciding what kind of exercise program is best for you.

There are essentially two different types of exercise, aerobic and anaerobic.

Aerobic exercise is called this because it encompasses the exercises that make you 'out of breath', so that you begin breathing more deeply as a way of replacing the depleted levels of oxygen in your body and blood. Aerobic exercise works your lungs and speeds up your heart, and it is therefore generally better at burning fat than is anaerobic exercise. Aerobic exercise takes in such things as running or jogging, swimming, cycling and even walking.

Anaerobic exercise on the other hand is the opposite, the kind of exercise that does not get you out of breath or makes you 'puff and pant'. Falling into this category would be the weightlifting. As previously suggested, anaerobic exercise does not burn off the fat as quickly as does aerobic, but it does have the benefit that it is more effective for speeding up your metabolism, leading to the effect of burning more calories even when at rest.

Aerobic exercise works as part of a fat burning weight loss plan, because your body normally turns to carbohydrates to provide the energy that you need. However, when exercising, your body starts to look to the stored fat to provide some of the necessary energy as well, hence the weight loss effect.

Anaerobic exercise on the other hand will generally be almost entirely fuelled by the carbohydrates in your body, and therefore the fat loss effect is far less noticeable. It does however have the advantage of speeding up your metabolism.

It is important to realize that there are situations where the two different forms of exercise tend to blur into one another. For example, if you start out walking slowly, then that is aerobic exercise, but if you start to push your speed until you reach jogging and then running pace, the expansion and contraction of your muscles means that you are also exercising anaerobically as well as aerobically.

**There are a couple more factors to bear in mind.**

Firstly, somewhat counter-intuitively, the heavier you are, the more calories you will burn. As you will see from the table in the next subsection, while a 120 pound person will burn fractionally over 9 cal per minute when jogging, a 180 pound person will use just short of 14 cal per minute doing exactly the same thing.

Secondly, even within a category of exercise, some forms of exercise are more effective for burning of fat than others. As an example, because of the effects of gravity, weight-bearing exercises such as jogging, running and walking are more effective for burning fat than would be non weight-bearing activities such as swimming or even cycling. In both of these cases, the effects of gravity have little or no influence on the amount of work you need to do.

No special equipment is needed, so no excuses…

Other important exercise considerations…

One thing that is often noticeable with people, who have not been exercising on a regular basis, is that they are mechanically inefficient. Even with walking, if you have not been walking in any serious way in the recent past, the chances are that you're walking 'style' and pattern is likely to be inefficient at first. Injuries and other physical damage are far more likely to happen in these early days, hence not trying to do too much, too soon.

Here is the most interesting thing about being mechanically inefficient in this way. Because you are expending energy on both the exercise that you are attempting to do and on making sure you do it properly, you will in fact burn more calories in these early days than you will later once you have acquired mechanical efficiency.

To get some idea of what I mean by mechanical efficiency, think of Olympic race walkers. Could you seriously consider walking 50 km at the speed that these people go at?

An Olympic 50 km race walking champion can do it because they are mechanically efficient. Despite the fact that they probably look slightly absurd to the untrained eye, with their hips swiveling, arms pumping and walking at a speed that falls marginally short of a jog, it's amazing to think that these people really do know what they are doing.

They do, because otherwise they would not be able to walk the distances they cover at the speeds that they achieve and maintain.

Now, I'm not suggesting that you adopt the walking style of an Olympic race walker, but you should appreciate that in the early days when you first start exercising, you are mechanically awkward. Consequently, you will burn more fat calories because you are fighting your inefficiency and exercising at the same time. It follows that the more you exercise the more efficient you will become and therefore the fewer calories you will burn.

I know that sounds a little unfair, but that is just the way it is.

In a similar way, you have already seen that the bigger you are, the more calories you are going to burn. It is therefore logical that as you lose the unwanted pounds and your weight starts to fall, you will again use fewer calories while exercising than you did at the beginning.

There is nothing that you can do about this, because it is something that happens which is unavoidable.

Another aspect of adopting an exercise program for the first time is realizing that it makes a difference to your life in many ways. For example, if you spend an hour or two in the gym every day, it is logical that you will be fairly exhausted. It would be no surprise if you found that you needed an afternoon nap, something that you had previously never considered.

During the time that you are sleeping, you are burning off the minimum number of calories, so to a certain extent, this will offset the benefits of the rigorous exercise that you have just undertaken.

If you put yourself through such a strenuous, vigorous exercise regime, it will probably increase your appetite too. It is not unknown for people who decide to exercise so vigorously to put on weight rather than lose it, because they are building muscle mass at the same time as eating far more than they were previously.

**Keep a journal…**

As soon as you start your fat weight loss program, the first thing that you must do is start a journal.

In this journal, record all of the exercise that you do, noting the type of exercise you have been doing, how long you are doing it for and the intensity of your activity.

For example, you can walk extremely slowly or you can walk at the speed of an Olympic race walker and there is going to be a significant difference between the calories you would burn off in these two alternative scenarios, so having a record of activity intensity is essential.

Remember that when you first exercising again, you are mechanically inefficient and heavy, and that the number of calories you're burning off is therefore larger.

On the other hand, as you become more used to regular exercise, you should be able to 'up' the intensity level so that you burn off the same number of calories as you did in the early days, or perhaps even more.

Don't forget to take this into account, and factor this in when you try to calculate a 'net calories burned' figure for recording in your journal.

You need to keep a constant record of your (declining) weight in this journal, plus a complete record of everything you eat and drink.

This journal will become your 'fat loss bible' over the coming weeks, and you should not underestimate the importance of keeping a journal of this nature because it can serve many positive purposes.

Firstly, there will be times when you will be tempted to skip an exercise session or tuck into a large bowl of ice cream with chocolate sauce. One quick glance at your journal should dissuade you from this (at least most of the time anyway!).

Secondly, I have no doubt that by following a regular program of exercise combined with eating and drinking in the way I recommend later in this manual, your weight will fall and you will become both slimmer and fitter.

When you are trying to lose weight, there is nothing more encouraging or inspiring than to see actual written proof that what you're trying to achieve is working, and do not forget the point I raised earlier about having a final target weight and sticking to it.

You should not realistically expect to see a massive weight loss every day unless you start off from being very obese indeed.

For this reason, I would not recommend that you take a note of your weight every day, but perhaps do so once or twice a week.

In this way, the weight loss becomes far more apparent, which is much more encouraging and far more likely to keep you going when temptation strikes from time to time (as it inevitably will).

**But I don't have time for exercise...**

Hogwash!

I understand that you are probably very busy every day of your life, but the fact is, everyone can make time for exercise if they apply some creative thinking and have enough determination to push through with what needs to be done.

For example, if you take the train, subway or bus to the office or factory every day, get off to three stops early and walk the rest of the way. It might add 10 minutes to your trip, but it will also provide the exercise that you must do if you are serious about shedding the fat.

In a similar way, if you use your own car to get to work, park it further away from the office if possible, and walk the rest of the way. If not, park on a lower level of the car park than you normally use, but use the stairs to get up to the floor you work on, rather than the elevator.

In fact, use the stairs whenever you can, because according to one sports nutrition expert, a person weighing 150 pounds will burn 12.5 calories per minute climbing stairs. If you work in an office block, use your break time or 15 minutes of your lunch to do some serious step climbing, and you will be making a significant impression on the 3500 calories that you have to burn to get rid of one pound of fat.

Perhaps you are a person who is extremely busy at work and equally busy at home with the family? You may even be a housewife or househusband, but there is still no excuse not to exercise.

For example, why not create a program of enjoyable exercise that the whole family can indulge in? Walking around the park, cycling or swimming together are all excellent exercise options and something that everyone can enjoy together. And, if you have children who are not yet able to swim, there is no better time to start teaching them than right now because swimming is a skill that could save their life one day.

**Here's another thought.**

Even everyday 'around the house' activities burn off the calories with washing the car, vacuuming the house, or digging the garden, all representing a form of activity and exercise.

So, if you usually take the car to a drive-through car wash every week, save yourself some money and get a workout every weekend by washing the car yourself.

If you vacuum the house or apartment once or twice a week, double the times that you do it. Not only will this make sure that you keep the house that much cleaner, which itself can have health benefits – cleaner air with less floating dust that can cause allergies – it will double the number of calories you burn doing basic housework as well.

If you have a garden, it could always be made to look neater and tidier couldn't it?

Once again, if you only 'do' the garden once a month, double up and double up the number of fat calories you are burning off at the same time.

**Water is the essence of life**

Water is the very essence of life.

You can live for a long time without food (protest hunger strikers have survived for over 10 weeks without anything to eat), but no-one can survive more than a few days without water.

Water serves many purposes for us. Your body uses water for moving the necessary nutrients to the places in your body that need them, and removes waste material from your body as well. It also helps the various organs in your body communicate with one another by providing a medium through which they can send electrical impulses to one another.

Here's a very important fact. A 5% reduction in bodily hydration will equate to a 20% fall in usable energy levels, which if you are exercising is a very serious consideration!

Water has zero calories, and as long as the water that you are drinking is alkaline water, it helps to offset the natural acidity of your body too.

The final factor about water is that when you drink it, it fills you up. This might sound simplistic, but you should pay a great deal of attention to this because when your stomach feels full, you don't want to eat.

Consequently, drinking plenty of water will naturally reduce the amount of food that you think you have to eat to overcome the feelings of hunger that you believe you are suffering.

You often see it quoted that you should drink eight glasses of water a day, but while this is a very reasonable starting point, the amount that you should drink as an individual depends upon your own metabolism.

Nevertheless, eight glasses of water a day would equate to somewhere around 3 to 4 liters, which is certainly a reasonable level of water to drink as a starting point, but if you want to drink more than this, then go for it – unless you drink the equivalent of a tanker truck of water, no harm will come of it, and it will add no calories.

Also, you have to be aware that your body often confuses hunger and thirst, because in both cases, your metabolism is calling out for something to fill an empty space in your stomach.

Hence, when you are on a diet, try drinking water every time you believe that you are hungry. Give it 15 minutes to see if the feeling of hunger persists, because the majority of the time, it won't, so water helps you to avoid taking in more calories than you need.

Before you sit down for a meal – indeed, if you're cooking at home, before you even start preparing or cooking the meal – drink at least one large glass of water, possibly two, depending on how long the preparation and cooking process takes. Once again, this will reduce the empty space in your stomach, make you feel less hungry and get rid of the temptation to nibble as you're going along or to try the food on numerous occasions during the cooking process.

For the same reason, drink at least two glasses of water when you first get out of bed in the morning. For most people, the time between dinner in the evening and breakfast is their longest period without food, so it is natural that you might feel especially hungry in the morning.

A couple of glasses of water will suppress your desire to eat and reduce the amount of food you are going to consume for breakfast.

Water is the most important fluid you can take in, and you should therefore try to replace as many as possible of the other drinks that you might take, with water. However, it is inevitable that there are times when you want to drink something other than water, in which case all you need to do is to seek some kind of sensible balance.

For example, if you drink ordinary tea or coffee, both contain caffeine which is a known diuretic. Consequently, for every cup of tea or coffee you drink, you should drink at least two glasses of water to replace lost fluids.

Similarly, some medicines and herbs also have diuretic qualities, so you need to drink sufficient water to replace those lost fluids.

Water helps to clean out your body and fill your stomach at the same time. Add this to the fact that it has absolutely no calories whatsoever, and you can understand why water should form an essential part of any sensibly planned natural weight loss program.

# Chapter 4- Go For A Healthy Meal Plan

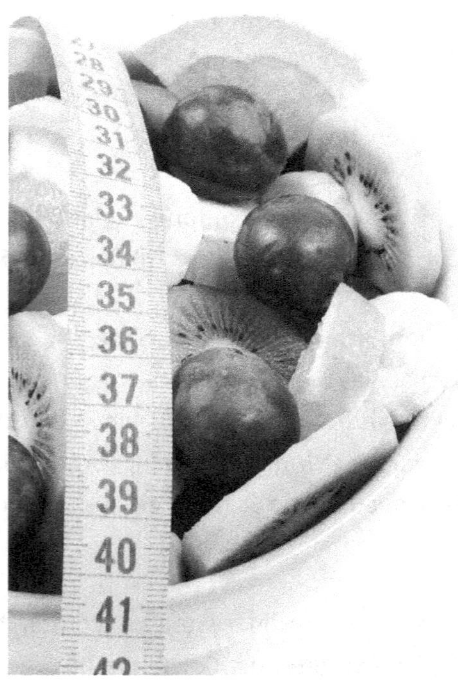

It's an unfortunate fact that the majority of us have a very dim (and unhealthy) view of vegetables, which is a shame because if you are trying to lose weight by shedding fat, the more vegetables you can include in your diet, the more effective you will be.

The fact is that vegetables are very high in nutrients and minerals, whereas they are very light in saturated fats and sugars, exactly the kind of things that you do not want to take in when you're trying to get rid of an excess of bodily fat.

There is really no limit on the amount of leafy green vegetables that you consume, while 'ordinary', day-to-day vegetables such as broccoli, Brussels sprouts, cauliflower and carrots are all a rich source of essential vitamins and nutrients.

There are many vegetables in the so-called 'Super Foods' list that you will find in 'Appendix A', so those are the ones to focus on.

Make it a point to eat a large green salad every day, including mustard or collard greens, kale, bok choy, cabbage, radish or spinach.

Also, find space for water filled vegetables such as cucumber and celery, because these have the double benefit of helping to keep you completely hydrated while adding very few additional calories to your diet.

The only thing that you have to place any limits on are starchy vegetables such as potatoes, beets, sweet potatoes and yams. Remember that these vegetables are primarily carbohydrates, so keep them separate from your proteins (meat, chicken etc).

A few portions of starchy vegetables every week should be enough, and when you eat them, try to do so earlier in the day because that gives your digestive system sufficient time to break these vegetables down before you go to bed.

As previously suggested, eating raw foods is a terrific way of boosting your fat loss efforts. If possible, you should aim to eat around about one pound of raw vegetables every day.

At the same time, there are some vegetables that are better cooked, but when you do so, make sure that they are steamed rather than boiled (boiling takes away a significant amount of the goodness), and of course, they should not be fried if at all possible!

**Eat More Fruit!**

Yes, I know that the chapter title is a bit abrupt but I cannot overemphasize how important fruits are as part of a sensibly structured fat reduction diet.

Fruits are packed with all the nutrients such as vitamins, minerals and fiber that you need to stay healthy and to lose the fat.

I have discovered that you should eat fruit in a certain way if you want to get the maximum benefit from it. The first thing is you should only eat ripe fruit, because the process of ripening is akin to human digestion. Hence, ripe fruit is already 'broken down' and really easy for your body to absorb the goodness from.

Secondly, you should eat ripe fruit on an empty stomach, giving it 30 to 45 minutes before you consume anything else. Doing things in this way means that you get the maximum benefit from the fruit that you have consumed, whereas if you eat fruit after a meal (for example), it will sit on the top of that food in your stomach and rot.

Follow your fruit with water, and you will have the maximum benefits from what you eaten and you will feel full before you start your next meal. Together, water and fruit act as a natural appetite suppressant, helping you to cut down on the amount of calories you are taking in.

You will find many fruits in the 'Super Foods' list, such as apples, bananas, blueberries and raspberries, so whichever of these most suit your tastes, go for it!

**Negative Calorie Foods**

The only truly zero calorie substance is water, but there are many foods that are listed as negative calorie foods.

This is because the process of digesting your food uses energy and therefore burns calories. Indeed, while your body is digesting your food, it is channeling most of your energy in that direction.

Negative calorie foods are those that do contain calories but in such small amounts that your body needs to use more calories to digest them than they contain. Hence, including a significant percentage of negative calorie foods in your everyday diet will inevitably provide a big boost for your fat loss efforts.

Other things to include in your diet

**Green tea**

It has long been believed that drinking green tea has many health giving benefits, amongst which is its ability to increase your metabolic rate - which raises the rate at which you are burning off calories.

In addition, it is also believed that it can help to enhance fat oxidization, which in turn helps your body to burn fat more quickly.

The secret weight loss weapons in green tea are catechin polyphenols, because while all teas contain antioxidants, it is only green tea that contains a significant amount of catechins.

These substances help to keep the weight off by blocking the normal movement of glucose sugars in the cells of your body. They also work in tandem with other substances in your body to increase the rate of fat oxidation, which is another way of saying that they help your body to burn fat as fuel rather than burning carbohydrates - which would normally be the 'first choice' fuel that your body would turn to.

The most abundant of the catechins found in green tea is epigallocatechin gallate (EGCG), which has the ability to alter hormone levels in the body which naturally helps to suppress your appetite. In addition, it is believed that it also affects the levels of noradrenaline which is a neurotransmitter that is partially responsible for controlling the levels of 'act ive' brown fat tissue in the body.

Strip away all of the science, and the net result is that drinking green tea or taking green tea extract is going to help to accelerate your fat loss while also helping to limit the further buildup of white fat tissue, the kind that you most want to get rid of.

I mentioned earlier that drinking water is vitally important, but if you want an alternative that you can drink from time to time which will also help to promote quicker fat loss, green tea is the answer you have been looking for.

**Acai berries**

Acai berries are small but nevertheless easily distinguishable purple/black berries that are originally from the Amazon rainforests. You will see that this is one of the foods mentioned on the 'Super Foods' list, as well it should be, because it is generally believed that there are a very wide range of health benefits to be gained from eating acai  berries or at least taking acai berry extract.

For example, it is suggested that acai can help to prolong your life, that it is a very powerful antioxidant and that it can help to keep your blood pressure under control as well.

However, in weight loss terms, the most important benefits are that acai helps boost energy levels and stamina, which should assist your exercise efforts.

In addition, because acai contain very high levels of dietary fiber, they will also help to prompt your digestive system to become more efficient, meaning that less 'junk' gets left in your stomach and digestive tract.

This is important, because most people do not take in sufficient dietary fiber in their normal diet. This means that over time, a significant amount of undigested food detritus gets left in your stomach (some claim that there can be up to 20 pounds of 'rubbish' in your gut that never gets shifted under normal circumstances).

As you drink lots more water while increasing your consumption of high fiber foodstuffs such as fruit, vegetables and acai, it is quite possible that you will see a very significant weight drop in the first few days as this accumulated 'junk' is flushed out of your system.

**Yerba Maté**

Yerba Maté is another plant that is indigenous to South America that is generally taken as a tea by steeping the leaves of the plant in boiling water (the drink is known as maté).

The weight loss related benefits of Yerba Maté are believed to be widespread, with claims that it can assist in burning fat, aid stamina and endurance, while helping to detoxify and 'clean out' your body.

However, probably the most important benefit to anyone who is trying to lose weight and burn fat is that Yerba Maté appears to be a very effective natural appetite suppressant. This helps you to follow a more sensible eating pattern.

**Apple cider vinegar**

Although it can have a bitter, sour taste, apple cider vinegar is a substance that is claimed to have a wide range of health benefits. While many of these benefits have not been tested or proven scientifically, a test conducted on 12 people in 2005 found that most of them reported feeling more full and satisfied after eating bread that had been infused with a few drops of apple cider vinegar when compared to eating the bread alone.

Hence, as with many other substances reported in this chapter, it appears that apple cider vinegar may act as a natural appetite suppressant, with many people taking it by mixing it with honey in a hot drink, or alternatively with fruit juice.

# Chapter 5- Comparison of Natural and Unnatural Fitness

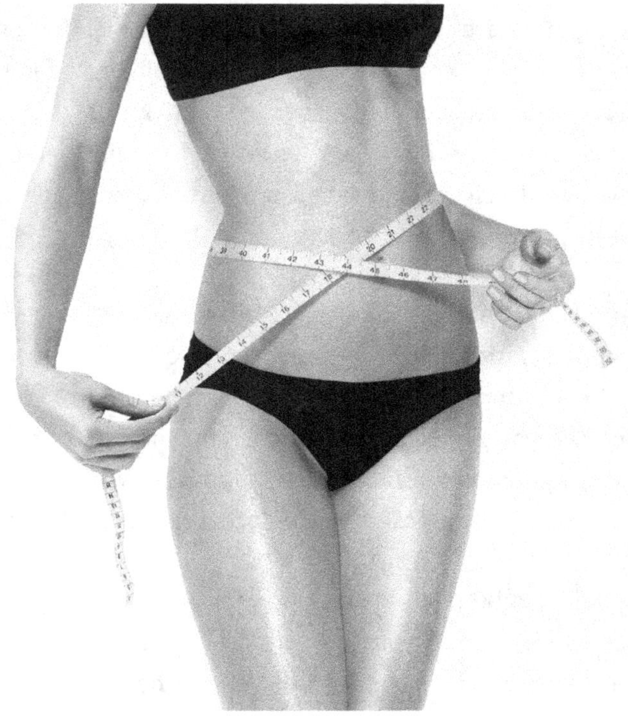

I already know two things about you. (1) You are an intelligent person (2) who has a weighty problem. I know that you are intelligent because you are seeking help to solve your problem and that is always the second step to solving a problem. The first one is acknowledging that there is, in fact, a problem that needs to be solved.

You need to lose some weight and it might surprise you to know that how much weight you need or want to lose is not an issue. It really doesn't much matter whether you need to lose 10 pounds; 110 pounds or more....the process for losing weight is exactly the same for every pound that must be lost. Not only is the process the same but the formula for losing a pound is the same as well. We will discuss the process and the formula later in this book.

You have no doubt discovered that there are as many weight loss 'experts' as there are weight loss programs. You can find programs and gurus that will swear that counting carbohydrates is the only way to go and you will find programs and gurus that promise counting fat grams is the only way to go. You can find calorie charts and carbohydrate charts and fat gram charts everywhere. Some of them are even free.

The truth of the matter is that, yes, you are going to have to count something.....calories, fat, carbohydrates...or with some plans 'points'. No matter...you will be counting something. We will be discussing the various counting options and then because you are an intelligent person you can choose for yourself what program will be the best one for you based on the facts that you will learn.

Here we will also be talking about ways to help you stay with your 'healthier eating plan' (never use the four letter word 'diet') long enough to learn how to manage your eating habits and thus your weight for the rest of your life.

Diet pills and physically altering surgeries are an option today. You have seen the 'miracles' of enormous weight loss by prominent people who have opted for these solutions. You will find out what those diet pills and surgeries are and the risks involved for opting for those solutions yourself.

**Natural Weight Loss**

Natural weight loss occurs when your body burns more energy than it is supplied with. What I mean by that is that food is the body's energy source. That is what the purpose of food is basically. Energy is measured in calories so I'm not advocating a calorie counting diet for you when I use the word 'calorie'.

The body burns that energy with every movement. Reach up and scratch your nose and you have burned some energy. Our bodies' burn energy even without movement. Our brains alone burn about 400 calories a day just thinking. We burn calories when we sleep.

If you ever watch sporting events, you might have heard sportscasters tell you that a participant in a bicycle race can lose up to 10 pounds just during the race and that is true. Some of that weight loss is fluid but most athletes know to replace lost fluid. Most of that weight loss that the sportscasters are talking about is actually caused by the body burning stored fat because the athlete is burning more energy than he is consuming.

Nobody reading this is likely to be one of those athletes who can burn 10 pounds of weight off while riding a bicycle, swimming or playing football but this is natural weight loss. Natural weight loss means burning more calories than are being consumed through food and drink over a 24 hour period without the aid of pills or surgical procedures.

There have been a lot of well publicized weight loss pills and pill combinations in recent years. Many have been proven to be unsafe for extended use while others have been proven to be downright deadly. When overweight patients ask their doctors for appetite suppressant pills, many times these doctors will quickly prescribe them and then fail to oversee their use or, even worse, they will fail to take their time to counsel their patients on the dangers of using these kinds of drugs.

It is very tempting to use diet pills in the quest for weight loss. Imagine the idea of just popping a little pill in and presto the weight is gone. Unfortunately, diet pills don't work like that. There really isn't a little magic pill. Unless a reduced calorie diet and exercise are used in conjunction with diet pills, the pills themselves will have no affect whatsoever on a person's weight.

Prescription diet pills as well as over-the counter diet pills all have side effects. These potential side effects certainly need to be weighed against any hoped for benefit to be derived from taking them.

Weight loss pills are usually appetite suppressants. Most of the prescription varieties have the potential for becoming habit forming all of them, prescription as well as over-the counter diet pills interfere with normal metabolism.

The Food and Drug administration has approved two drugs for use as diet pills. They are sold under different brand names, of course, but there really are only two drugs. They are orlistat and sibutramine. Sibutramine is sold as Meridia and Orlistat is sold as Xenical. Sibutramine is an appetite suppressant. Orlistat is a lipase inhibitor, which means it interferes with the body's ability to absorb fat.

All prescription diet pills have one or the other ingredient....either orlistat or sibutramine. If your doctor prescribes a diet pill for you, you need to be aware of the possible side effects that the drugs can cause.

The makers of Meridia (Sibutramine) list these side effects on their website:

If you experience any of the following serious side effects, stop taking Meridia and seek emergency medical attention or contact your doctor immediately:

•an allergic reaction (difficulty breathing; closing of your throat; swelling of your lips, tongue, or face; or hives);

•an irregular heartbeat;

•high blood pressure (severe headache, blurred vision); or

•seizures.

The makers of Xenical (Orlistat) list these side effects on their website: "More common side effects may include: Abdominal discomfort or pain, anxiety, arthritis, back pain, diarrhea, dizziness, earache, fatigue, fatty or oily stools, fecal urgency or incontinence, flu, gas with fecal discharge, gum problems, headache, increased defecation, menstrual problems, muscle pain, nausea, oily discharge, rectal discomfort or pain, respiratory tract infections, skin rash, sleep problems, tooth problems, urinary tract infections, vaginal inflammation, vomiting"

OK...you say maybe diet pills aren't the way to go. Those side effects sound gross and maybe even dangerous.

There are many surgeries available for very obese people. These surgeries cause the body to not function as it was designed to function and thus they produce weight loss. There are basically three types of surgeries performed for the purpose of the patient losing weight:

• Reduction of the size of the stomach. This procedure simply reduces the physical size of the stomach by stapling or other methods and makes it impossible for the patient to consume much food at a meal.

• Removal of a portion of the intestines. This procedure removes a portion of the intestine and thus reduces the amount of intestine that comes into contact with food consumed by the patient.

• Reduction of the size of the stomach AND Removal of a portion of the intestines.

There are several different names for these types of bariatric surgeries. You can read about the potential risks here. There are many risks associated with bariatric surgeries. Just the first five of those listed are:

• Bleeding from a tear to the liver, spleen, or blood vessels

• Bowel obstruction, requiring further surgery

• Cardiac problems. Greatest risk in patients who are the most overweight, or who have cardiac disease

• Complications due to anesthesia and medications.

• Deep vein thrombosis. Blood clots in the large leg veins. They become serious when they float up into the blood vessels of the lungs.

Sometimes bariatric surgeries are required for those who are more than 100 pounds overweight and have serious weight related health problems but bariatric surgery should never be entered into lightly. The risks are great.

Diet pills can be tempting but they won't work at all unless a reduced calorie diet is followed and exercise is increased. Bariatric surgeries are sometimes necessary but should not ever be considered if there is an alternative of losing weight naturally.

Unnatural weight loss means burning more calories than are consumed over a 24 hour period with the aid of diet pills or surgeries.

## Food Consumption Affects Weight Loss

The first thing that you need to know is that 1 pound of body weight is equal to 3500 calories. If you gain a pound that means that you consumed 3500 calories more than you burned. If you lose a pound that means that you have burned 3500 calories more than you consumed. That figure does not change whether the calories are consumed from fat or carbohydrates or whether they were burned by riding a bicycle, swimming or just verging out in front of the TV. A calorie is a calorie is a calorie. This is important information in your quest for weight loss and weight control so make note of it.

1 pound of body weight gained or lost = 3500 calories.

The trick to losing weight is to eat fewer calories AND burn more calories each day. That is the basis that all 'diets' (there is that four letter word again) are based upon no matter whether you are counting calories, fat grams of carbohydrates.

Even though you may believe that most of the calories that your body burns in a day are from the exercise that you do, you are not right. Only about 30% of the calories you burn each day are from exercise. However, the exercise that you do can influence at what rate you burn calories when you are not exercising. Exercise or the lack of exercise affects your metabolic rate....that is, the rate at which your body burns calories when it is at rest. About 60% of the calories that you burn each day are burned when you are not engaging in physical exercise.

The body burns calories to fuel the thousands of chemical reactions required to maintain body temperature, repair cells and keep your heart, lungs, liver and kidneys functioning.

So, you ask, where do the other 10% of the calories get burned up? 30% during exercise, 60 % the rest of the time....what about the other 10%? Those are the ones that the body uses to actually digest the food you eat that supplies all of the calories needed for everything else.

There is more. All calories are not created equally. Our bodies simply do not process all calories consumed in exactly the same way.

Calories that are consumed in the form of Essential Fatty Acids (EFAs), for example, contain about 9 calories per gram but our bodies don't use those calories as an energy source. These calories are used to rebuild cells and tissues, particularly after an injury. If consumed at very high levels they increase metabolic rate and increase fat burn off, resulting in loss of weight. (This is the basic theory of the Dr. Atkins Diet). Consumption of high levels of EFAs has been linked to heart disease but that is an on-going debate in the scientific community.

More calories are absorbed from refined foods because it takes so much longer for them to pass through our systems. Natural and unrefined food (an apple for example) usually takes between 12 and 15 hours to pass through our digestive systems. Refined foods can take up to 75 hours to pass through our digestive systems and our systems continue to extract calories from them for the whole 75 hours.

Our bodies require vitamins and minerals to properly digest food therefore empty calorie foods....those that contain no vitamins or minerals.....are stored as fat while our bodies wait for the needed vitamins and minerals to properly process them.

Each human being is unique. All human bodies do not process not use calories in the exact same way. You know at least one of those people who can eat like the proverbial horse and never gain a pound....they make my eyes turn green with envy. Then we all know those people (we may be them) who can just think about eating a donut and gain a couple of pounds. It hardly seems fair but that is just the way it is.

We each have to learn what and how much we can eat in order to lose those unwanted pounds. We can use the available charts to help guide our choices but when it comes right down to it, each of us will have to determine what and how much of it is the right thing for ourselves.

**Exercise Affects Weight Loss**

It shouldn't come as a big surprise to anybody that you are burning more energy when you are standing than when you are sitting, more energy when you are walking than when you are standing and more energy when you are running than when you are walking. That is just common sense.

When you begin your 'eating healthier' plan, you really need to include an exercise plan to go along with it. You can only eat just so many fewer calories than you burn each day and exercise allows you to burn more for the time you are exercising plus increase your metabolic rate for several hours after you are through exercising. In addition, vigorous physical exercise causes our brains to produce dandy little hormones called endorphins that lift our moods and make us feel happier.

# Chapter 6- Low Fat Diets, Low Carb Diets & Low Calorie Diet

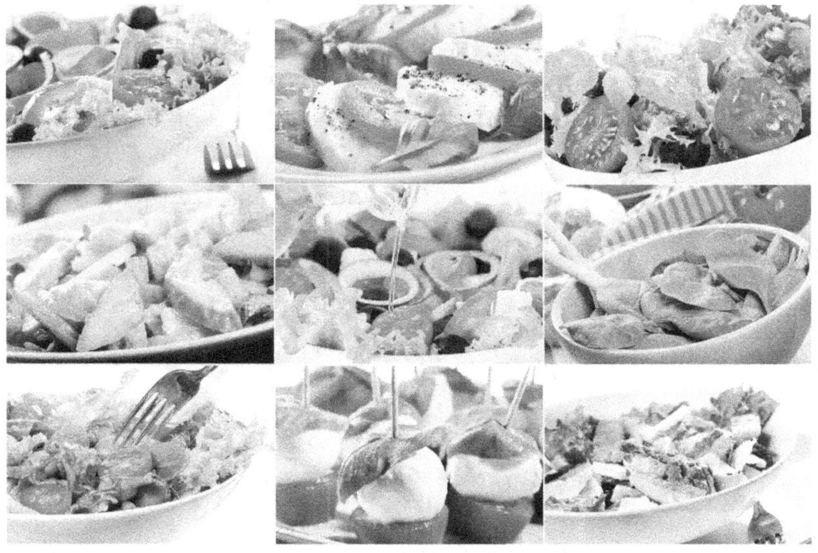

Let me begin this chapter be saying that SOME fat is essential in our diets to help our bodies absorb fat soluble vitamins like Vitamin A and to supply two types of essential fatty acids (EFAs) that our bodies need but don't produce.

Many people claim that their diets are absolutely fat free but that is virtually impossible. Foods that are labeled 'fat free' still contain up to ½ gram of fat per serving and there is some fat in all fruit, vegetables, and grains. Skim milk is not fat free, either. While it is possible to eat a low fat diet it is impossible to eat a no fat diet.

Actually calculating how many grams of fat that you should consume in a day in order to lose weight sounds like you need a degree in higher mathematics but maybe it isn't quite as hard as it sounds. The entire process begins with the number of calories that you intend to eat in the first place. When you determine that number then you must calculate the number of grams of fat that you have consumed in a day (each gram contains 9 calories) and multiply by 9. Divide that number by the number of calories that you have consumed. Now, you multiply that answer by 100 and you will have arrived at the percentage of fat calories contained in your diet. You need to aim for a fat gram consumption that equals 20-30% of your total caloric consumption. You can find calorie and fat gram charts on the Internet and in real world book stores.

You can also find resources on the Internet that can help you to effectively substitute one food for another and thereby decrease your fat intake. Some handy substitutions are:

• Use 1 cup of applesauce rather than 1 cup of butter or oleo in baking

• Use 8 ounces of yogurt rather than 8 ounces of cream cheese

• Use 4 cups low fat stock, fruit juice or wine for sautéing rather than 1 cup of oil. Sauté until all of the liquid evaporates.

• Use 2 egg whites instead of 1 whole egg

• Ground turkey rather than ground beef

• Low fat frozen yogurt rather than ice cream

• Canadian bacon, turkey bacon or lean ham rather than bacon

Remember that the object of a low fat diet is LOW fat and not NO fat. Also remember that if you are counting fat grams you will also be counting calories.

A low fat diet is considered one of the healthiest diets. It is one that is recognized by the American Heart Foundation as well as by the American Medical Association.

A low fat diet is considered very beneficial for heart patients and for those with diabetes or at risk for stroke or heart attack.

Those who follow low fat diets have lowered their blood pressure as well as lost weight and both are very good things.

Conclusion: Low fat diets will product weight loss mainly because they are reduced caloric diets, as well.

**Low Carb Diets**

The first low-carb diet broke onto the weight loss scene in 1972 and changed the world's beliefs about dieting forever. According to the Dr. Atkins diet plan a person could eat all of the protein and fat that they wanted....there was no limit. Have a dozen eggs scrambled in a whole stick of butter and an entire pound of bacon for breakfast.....just NO toast or bread of any kind....no orange juice either.

JUST protein. For lunch have a whole pig and for dinner have a whole cow...just no vegetables, no bread, no potatoes, no rice, no pasta, nothing that contained sugar or starch in any form. America said, "WOW! You mean we don't have to live on 500 calories a day and eat nothing but lettuce, boiled eggs and grapefruit?" The Dr. Atkins Diet became all the rage and the diet world quickly learned three important things:

1. All calories are not created equal.

2. Eliminating carbohydrates from a diet causes weight loss.

3.      A high protein diet produces the worst case of halitosis (bad breath) in the universe and breath mints are not on the Dr. Atkins Diet plan.

The medical community was appalled. Doctors just knew that all that saturated fat was certain to cause major health problems....and the battle lines were drawn. The benefits and risks of the Atkins Diet still rages today.

Recent research results suggest that the high protein, high fat, low carbohydrate diet does not cause serious health concerns about an increased heart attack or stroke risk. Abdominal cramping caused by the lack of dietary fiber and bad breath are the most commonly reported side effects of the Dr. Atkins diet.

Dr. Atkins died at age 72 from head injuries sustained when he slipped on an icy sidewalk. At his death he weighed 258 pounds and was six feet tall....a height and weight combination that is considered to be obese. He had several heart attacks and suffered from heart disease. His wife and others claim that the weight was due to bloating and that the heart disease was the result of a viral infection.

Dr. Atkins did make changes to his diet plan between the time it was first published in the 1970's and the latest edition that was published in 2002. He recommended a reduction in the consumption of red meat but that fact was never widely publicized.

The Dr. Atkins Diet Revolution book can be purchased in book stores and online. It remains one of the bestselling books of all time.

**The South Beach Diet**

Dr. Arthur Agatston designed The South Beach Diet in the mid 1990's. Dr. Agatston is a cardiologist and was concerned with the high fat diet Dr. Atkins diet plan than many of his patients were following. He believed that the 20 grams of carbohydrates that were recommended in the Dr. Atkins diet plan was too low. He recommends 30 to 40 grams of carbohydrate consumption each day and insists that there is a difference between kinds of carbohydrates. He divides carbohydrates into 'simple carbohydrates' and 'complex carbohydrates' and asks dieters to choose the complex carbohydrate variety.

Some foods that contain simple carbohydrates and should be avoided according to the South Beach Diet are:

• Table Sugar

• Cakes

• Biscuits

• Jam

• Chocolate

• Candy

• Honey

• Soft Drinks

Some foods that contain complex carbohydrates and are allowed in moderate quantities on the South Beach Diet are:

• Pasta

• Brown Rice

• Potatoes

• Turnips

• Carrots

• Whole wheat bread

• Whole grain cereals

• Corn

• Yams

• Peas

• Beans

You can find a good list of foods and their carbohydrate values here. The South Beach diet has proven itself to be popular, as well as, effective providing the dieter limits portion sizes and chooses complex carbohydrates rather than simple carbohydrates.

One of the most famous South Beach Dieters is former President Bill Clinton.

**The Zone Diet**

The Zone diet was developed by Barry Sears, Ph.D. He is not a medical doctor or a dietician. He is a biochemist. His theory is that if a person eats the correct ratio of carbohydrates (40%) to protein (30%) to fat (30%), their hormonal balance will be established and thus their health, weight and athletic performance will be maximized. They will be in 'the zone'....hence, the name.

The basic concepts of the Zone diet are that the dieter is to eat small meals frequently...no more than 5 hours between meals and foods such as sweets, chips and junk food are eliminated while foods such as grapefruit, nuts and lentils are increased.

The food plans in the Zone diet average between 1200 and 1300 calories per day for an average size woman. Since most women would lose weight on that daily caloric intake, the diet does work.

Dr. Sears (biochemist) makes some clinically unsubstantiated claims as to health benefits produced by the Zone diet. His claims of more efficient fat burning and reduced incidences of disease are unproven. Dr. Sears blames insulin resistance as the cause of all obesity and there is clear scientific evidence that this is simply not the case.

However, even though Dr. Sears' conclusions are seriously flawed, the diet does in fact produce weight loss. It does so because it is a low calorie diet and the meal recommendations are balanced. It will do you no harm. If you choose to follow the Zone diet, by all means do so, and just remember that most of the hype is.....well....hype.

Conclusion: There are many versions of the low carb diet. I have listed only three of them here. The body deals with carbohydrates derived from protein in a different way than it does those derived from carbohydrates. Low carb diets work but one needs to be aware of health concerns related to prolonged consumption of foods high in saturated fats.

**Less Calorie Diets**

I remember years ago when my mother would go on a diet. She would live for weeks at a time on nothing but lettuce, boiled eggs and black coffee. There weren't many diet foods on the market back then apparently. The first 'diet' soft drink was introduced by Coke in 1963. It was called 'Tab'. Since then the diet food industry has exploded. You can find reduced calorie, reduced fat, no fat, low carb, reduced carb etc. etc. etc. on the shelves and in the coolers of every grocery store in America.

The sad obesity statistics are that there are 58 Million Overweight; 40 Million Obese; 3 Million morbidly Obese and it isn't getting any better. The number of overweight children in America tripled in less than 30 years. Most of those who are overweight are on some kind of weight loss diet....apparently these diets aren't working wonders.

We have counted fat grams and carb grams. We have eaten low fat, no fat, low carb and no carb and yet we are still the most obese nation on the face of the planet. It seems that no matter what kind of diet comes into vogue weight control always boils back down to calories consumed versus calories expended, doesn't it?

You can find advice by the ton on the Internet and in every book store in every strip mall in America on weight loss. Still, when you take out all of the hype losing weight means that you must consume fewer calories each day than you burn.

You've most likely guessed by now that I am not a big fan of higher mathematics but I can add and subtract. I'll bet you can, too. On a good day, I can even balance my checkbook so here is a simple mathematical formula to determine how many calories you can consume in a day and maintain your weight based on your height:

Start with 1000 calories for your first 5 feet of height and add 100 calories for each inch of height over 5 feet. If you are 5 feet 5 inches tall, you can have 1500 calories a day to maintain your weight. That wasn't hard, was it?

Now for some more math. In order to lose 1 pound of body weight you must reduce your caloric intake by 3500 calories. To lose 1 pound of body weight in a week's time that means that you must reduce your caloric intake by about 500 calories a day....OR expend 500 more calories in exercise a day....OR a combination of both reducing calorie intake AND increasing caloric expenditures by exercising more that totals a 500 calorie reduction.

If you are a woman who is 5'5" tall using a combination of reduced caloric consumption and increased caloric expenditure, this means that you will consume 1250 calories a day and do about 40 minutes of aerobic exercise a day for a week and lose 1 pound of body weight. These calculations are based on the average.

They are not hard and fast rules. We aren't like check books or ATM machines. What goes in versus what comes out is not set in stone. Each of us is different and our metabolisms are different. Some of our bodies burn calories more efficiently than others.

You can find many reduced calorie diets that include meal plans for diets of various daily caloric values each day beginning with a 1000 calorie daily diet plan through a 2000 calorie daily diet plan. These plans are available through your private physician's offices, on the Internet and in most places that sell books.

There is a free online calorie counter available here. You do need to remember that calories are based on the size of the portion, however. We will discuss portion control later in this e-book.

Today packaged foods are labeled with calorie, fat and carbohydrate content. It hasn't always been like that but thanks to new labeling laws this information is required to be put right there on the labels where we can read it. Remember, though, that the totals are usually listed PER SERVING and above that is information telling you just what a serving consists of. Most of the time the serving size is listed as ½ cup or 1 cup but sometimes the serving size is listed in ounces.

You can find liquid diet plans, as well. Slim Fast was the first but it has a lot of competition out there on grocery store shelves now days. Most of these liquid meals contain about 300 calories each which means that you can replace all three daily meals with a liquid meal and have a few saltine crackers each day to consume only 1000 calories a day. Most of these liquid diet plans suggest that you use them to replace only one or two meals each day.

The single most important thing that you can do in order to gain control over your weight, however, is to learn about food. Learn what foods contain sugars and starches, which foods contain protein and fat.

A healthy diet isn't a 'diet' at all. It is a healthier way of eating that you can stick to long enough to lose the weight you need to lose and when you reach your goal weight you will know enough about food and how your body reacts to it so that you can maintain your weight loss for life.

Conclusion: Low fat and low carb diets are still low calorie diets. It takes eating fewer calories that you burn to lose weight. Weight can be lost through eating less and exercising more.

**Diet Programs**

It seems every time I turn on the television lately there is another advertisement for a weight loss system that is guaranteed to change my life and be absolutely painless to boot. It has, however, been my experience that nothing is easy OR painless when it comes to losing weight. Some ways are less painful than others though and we can all use all of the help we can get.

Here I will review some of the better known weight loss programs...ones that have at least been around for awhile. All of these programs can be considered natural weight loss programs because they do not advocate diet pills or bariatric surgeries.

**NutriSystem**

It has been more than 30 years since NutriSystem was founded and it has since proven that it does have staying power. The NutriSystem program consists of prepackaged meals and unlimited consultations with weight loss councilors.

For many years there was no means provided by NutriSystem for their customers to communicate with each other. Now there are message boards provided on the Internet where members can post their success stories and exchange information and ideas with other NutriSystem customers.

The prepackaged meals that are provided are nutritionally balanced. About 55% of the calories in these prepackaged meals come from carbohydrates, 25% come from protein and about 20% come from fat.

There are prepackaged meals that are designed for men, women, children, type II diabetics and vegetarians. There is, additionally, an incentive program to get a free week's supply of meals if the patron orders and pays for a month's supply online.

There is no membership fee and there are no dues. The only cost is the prepackaged meals. At this writing the cost for the meals was about $280 per month. A month of packaged meals consists of:

28 breakfasts

28 lunches

28 dinners and...

28 snacks/desserts

The biggest advantage of the NutriSystem program is that it removes all food making decisions. The portions are controlled and there is the convenience factor to consider.

The biggest disadvantages are that the NutriSystem meals are rather expensive and there is little education about food and lifestyle changes provided.

**Diet Center**

The Diet center has been around quite awhile, too…almost 30 years now. I had a little trouble deciding whether to include them in this report and call them a natural weight loss program but I finally decided that since they do not advocate the use of diet pills or bariatric surgeries they do qualify as a natural weight loss program.

There are two programs offered by the Diet center. They are:

1. Exclusively You- Personalized Diet Plan

When you enroll in the Exclusively You Diet Plan you receive free: 1 wk of Multi-Vitamin Supplement

1 wk of Anti-Oxidant Formula 1 wk of the Cal-Mag Formula 2 Instant Shape-Up Shakes

2 Instant Shape-Up Bars

In order to continue with the program, a patron is required to purchase additional kits for $14.95 each. Each kit contains a week's supply of the vitamin supplement, the anti-oxidant formula and the Cal-Mag formula.

2. Instant Shape Up

When you enroll in the Instant Shape Up plan you receive free: 2 week supply of chewable diet supplements

2 week supply of new Fiber Capsules

In order to continue with the program, a patron is required to purchase additional Shape Up kits at $19.95 per two week supply.

On their website, the Diet Center provides a 16 week program that includes, weigh-in reminders, diet plans, meal plans, recipes, dieting information and a member's forum. The cost of the 16 week program is $96.

Out in the real brick and mortar world, when you visit a Diet Center, buy the above listed supplements and join their program, you receive daily weigh-ins and one-on- one counseling, as well as, dieting guides and meal plan assistance.

The main problem that I have with Diet Center is the heavy reliance on supplements. Not that supplements can't help because they can. They just should not be used as a replacement for information about the relationship between food and weight. Also, I found that the Diet Center plans did not emphasis the importance of physical exercise to weight loss and weight control.

That said, the Diet Center program does recommend a balanced natural diet and does not advocate the use of diet pills or bariatric surgeries in their weight loss programs so, if you think that the Diet Center can offer you the assistance you need for natural weight loss, by all means contact them.

**Health Management Resources**

Health Management Resources® has been in existence for about 20 years. The HMR approach to weight is loss is the use of a very low calorie diet with the use of low calorie shakes or entrees as meal replacements. Their specialty is the very fast loss of a significant amount of weight. Health Management Resources is associated with the Mayo Clinic and expense of the diet is often covered by health insurance providers.

Participants in the Health Management Resources program are required to attend weekly meetings that last about an hour and a half. These classes are designed to teach the specifics of weight loss and weight management.

Participation in the Health Management Resources 'Very Low Calorie Diet' (VLCD) requires the written approval of the participant's personal physician. There are no exceptions.

I looked for but could not find the price for the shakes that are included in the program requirements. The cost of 11 entrees is $39.50 plus a shipping charge of $9.95.

This is a direct quote taken from the Health Management Resources website:

"HMR® weight loss foods should not be used as a sole source of nutrition without medical approval. These products are not to be used without medical supervision if total daily calorie intake is less than 800 calories. These products are not intended for use by infants, children, or pregnant and lactating women. Consult a physician before starting any diet."

*Eat and Live Healthy*

There is no doubt that the HMR® program does produce very rapid weight loss. The problems that I see with the program are that there is a very heavy commitment to exercise required (burning 2000 calories per day through vigorous physical activity), the use of prepackaged foods and shakes that are on the pricy side and the possibility of problems with an intolerance to cold, dizziness and headache caused by such a low calorie diet.

**Jenny Craig**

You can't call Jenny Craig ® the new kid on the block exactly but in relation to other weight loss programs they are relatively new. The Jenny Craig weight loss program began in Australia in 1983. Neither Jenny nor her Australian born husband, Sidney Craig had any formal training in nutrition, yet they developed a weight loss program that eventually developed into a multi-million dollar weight loss company.

The advertisements say that the Jenny Craig ® weight loss program is based on healthy eating, self-awareness and exercise and those claims do seem to be substantiated.

The prepackaged meals that must be purchased by patrons are balanced. They are 60 % carbs-20% fat-20% protein. These prepackaged meals do help patrons with the problem of portion control and they are, without a doubt, very convenient.

Patrons have weekly consultations with coaches. These coaches are not formally trained dieticians but rather they are trained by the Jenny Craig Company. Their purpose is to track the progress of the patrons, assist in changing old habits, teach new skills, and help patrons to stay motivated.

Physical exercise is promoted and rather enthusiastically. Patrons are encouraged to increase their physical activity and instructed about how to get the most out of a half hour of daily exercise.

The Jenny Craig program offers a membership for $49 to lose all the weight a patron wants to lose....the $49 does not include the required prepackaged meals. These prepackaged meals cost between $11 and $15 dollars per day...which is a little more than what most other programs cost.

Jenny Craig does offer a transitional program to help patrons go from eating the prepackaged, portion controlled meals to eating meals that they prepare at home or eat out in restaurants once they have reached their desired weight goals.

The only real problems that I see with the Jenny Craig weight loss program is the lack of support between members and, of course, the high price of the prepackaged meals that patrons are required to purchase.

In the world of weight loss companies, I would rate Jenny Craig as one of the good guys of the industry. Pricy but good.

Conclusion: The diet programs listed here are only the tip of the iceberg. The weight loss industry is a crowded place and new programs surface daily. The fact is that these programs offer nothing that a dieter could not accomplish on their own if they were motivated. They do, however, offer a way for a dieter to jump start their weight loss program. No weight loss program, particularly one that advocated a very low calorie consumption, should be started without the consent of your personal physician.

# Chapter 7- The Importance of Keeping a Healthy Fitness Diet

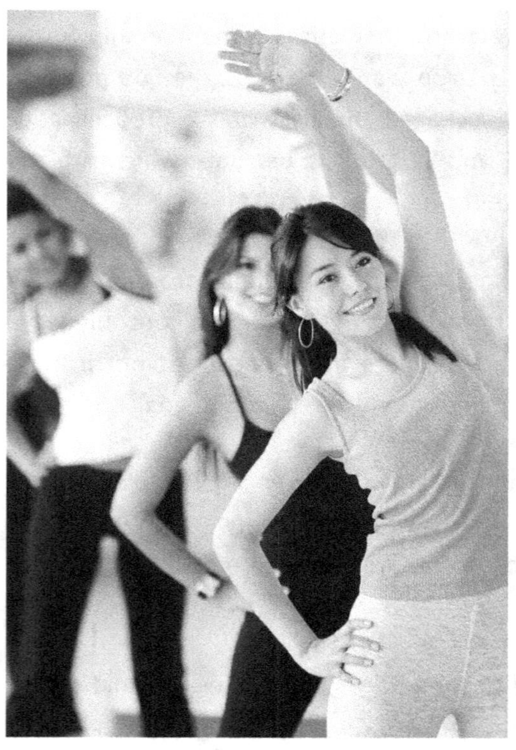

Our attitudes and beliefs about the consumption of food and its relationship to weight is something that we all learned at the family dinner table in our formative years. Those ideas and the habits that were formed came early into our lives and they are coming early into the lives of our children and our grandchildren. Food consumption ideas and habits seem to be passed down from generation to generation, don't they? There are exceptions, of course, but have you ever noticed that whole families either tend to be of normal weight, below normal weight, or obese? Part of that is genetics, no doubt, but part of it is caused by the food consumption habits that are passed down through families.

It is a fact that America is the fattest nation on earth. Not one single 'expert' disputes it. We are an obese nation. In America today there are 58 Million people who are Overweight, 40 Million people who are Obese and 3 Million people who are morbidly Obese. Those numbers are scary, for sure, but that isn't even the worst of the problem.

An even worse part of the American obesity problem is that we are raising obese kids. A whopping 13% of American children five years of age and younger are obese. It gets worse.

The following statistics were taken from Heart Check at the American Heart Association website:

**Overweight Children AHA Recommendation**

Overweight children are more likely to be overweight adults. Successfully preventing or treating overweight in childhood may reduce the risk of adult overweight. This may help reduce the risk of heart disease and other diseases.

When defining overweight in children and adolescents, it's important to consider both weight and body composition.

Among American children ages 6–11, the following are overweight, using the 95th percentile or higher of body mass index (BMI) values on the CDC 2000 growth chart:

• For whites (only), 11.9 percent of boys and 12.0 percent of girls.

• For blacks or African Americans (only), 17.6 percent of boys and 22.1 percent of girls.

• For Mexican Americans, 27.3 percent of boys and 19.6 percent of girls.

Among adolescents ages 12–19, the following are overweight, using the 95th percentile or higher of BMI values on the CDC 2000 growth chart:

• For whites (only), 13.0 percent of boys and 12.2 percent of girls.

• For blacks or African Americans (only), 20.5 percent of boys and 25.7 percent of girls.

• For Mexican Americans, 27.5 percent of boys and 19.4 percent of girls.

Obesity is reaching epidemic proportions in America. We can't do anything about what other families do, of course, but we can take control of our own family's eating habits. We can learn about the relationship of food consumption to weight and pass that information along to our own children and our grandchildren. It might just be our greatest legacy.

**Obesity Affects Us Physically**

The truth is that obesity is at least as dangerous to our health and the health of our families as smoking. No sane parent would ever serve cigarettes up to their children but these same otherwise responsible and intelligent parents will serve up meals that are high in fat and low in nutrients. Big Macs and fries are not home cooked meals but it seems that most of today's kids think of them that way.

Obesity causes a 50% to 100% increase in mortality rates for all reasons. White men between the ages of 20 and 30 with a BMI

(Body Mass Index) of 45 will shorten their life expectancy by 13 years. Obese white women between the ages of 20 to 30 with a BMI of 45 can expect to die 8 years sooner than if they were of average weight.

Many common human diseases are said to be 'obesity related'. The dictionary defines an Obesity-related disease as: "Any disease for which obesity is a significant risk factor." Some such obesity related diseases are:

Type II Diabetes: Type II Diabetes is sometimes referred to as insulin-resistant diabetes, non-insulin dependent diabetes, and adult-onset diabetes. Obesity is considered to be one of the main risk factors for the onset of Type II Diabetes by all leading medical authorities.

Hypertension: (High Blood Pressure) About 75% of cases of hypertension is linked directly to obesity. There are many theories as to why obesity is such a high factor in the causes of hypertension and there has even been debate about whether the hypertension and obesity should even be classified as two different problems.

Stroke: There are three causes for a stroke. They are:

• Clogging of arteries within the brain (e.g. lacunar stroke)

• Hardening of the arteries leading to the brain (e.g. carotid artery occlusion)

• Embolism to the brain from the heart or an artery

The first two of these listed causes are directly related to obesity. The fat in the blood stream attaches itself to artery walls where it hardens and reduces blood flow.

Heart Attack: These are many factors associated with the cause of a heart attack. Obesity is one of the major ones. Obesity raises the risk of heart disease and, thus, heart attacks, because it's associated with high cholesterol levels, high blood pressure and diabetes, not to mention all of the additional living flesh that must be supplied with oxygen carrying blood that must be pumped by the heart.

Cancer: Some forms of cancer are directly related to obesity. Obesity is thought to be a major contributing factor in breast cancer, cancer of the prostate, cancer of the rectum and cancer of the colon, for example.

Gallbladder Disease: Obesity is a major contributing factor to the onset of gallbladder disease. Some studies in animals suggest that saturated fats and refined sugars are the culprits but most studies conclude that obesity itself is the problem and not specific foods. According to the American Obesity Association, "Gallstones are common among overweight and obese persons. Gallstones appear in persons with obesity at a rate of 30% versus 10% in non-obese."

Gout: Obesity causes an increase in the production of uric acid and a decrease in the amount of elimination from the body. This causes the deposit of uric acid crystals in joints and tissue and causes what we call gout.

Osteoarthritis: Osteoarthritis of the hand, hip, back and especially the knee is directly linked to obesity. A weight loss of only 10 to 15 pounds has been proven to relieve the symptoms and delay the progress of the disease.

Rheumatoid Arthritis has been found to be directed related to obesity in both men and women, as well.

Birth Defects: Maternal obesity has been linked to an increased incidence of neural tube defects in newborns.

Carpal Tunnel Syndrome: The risk is about four times higher for a person developing Carpal Tunnel Syndrome if they are obese. Obesity was found to be a larger risk factor for the development of Carpal Tunnel Syndrome than repetitive motion or a workplace activity. In a recent study of the disease, more than 70% of the test subjects were obese.

Renal Disease: According to the American Obesity Association, "Obesity may be a direct or indirect factor in the initiation or progression of renal disease, as suggested in preliminary data."

Liver Disease: Obesity is as much of a contributing factor of liver disease as alcohol abuse. Obesity is the major factor for nonalcoholic steatohepatitis.

Body Pain: Those who are obese have body pain more often and it is much more acute than those of normal weight. Joint pain and foot pain are reported more often by the obese.

Pancreatitis: Those patients who are obese with Pancreatitis develop significantly more complications, including respiratory failure, than non-obese patients.

Sleep Apnea: Upper body obesity is the most significant factor for obstructive sleep apnea. Sixty to Seventy percent of those with obstructive sleep apnea are obese.

The above list of obesity related diseases is only a partial one. These are many other diseases that are either caused by or made worse by obesity.

Does depression cause obesity or does obesity cause depression? That question is much like the age old 'which came first....the chicken or the egg' question. The fact is, though, that depression, as well as anxiety is much more prevalent in those who are obese than either are in the general population. Obesity can and does cause low self-esteem which in and of itself can cause many mental and emotional problems.

While I am certainly not minimizing the mental and emotional problems that obesity can cause for adults, these problems are many times larger for obese children.

Adults generally refrain from making cruel and cutting remarks to obese adults but children are blunt and sometimes even cruel when it comes to other children who are obese.

When I speak of 'depression' here, I am not talking about the common garden variety depression that all of us experience from time to time. Those 'blue' days that just happen, and sometimes for no apparent reason, happen to everybody.

Deep clinical depression is a different thing altogether. Clinical depression doesn't just last for a few hours or even for just a day or for a few days. It moves in lock, stock and barrel and it stays.

The dictionary defines 'Clinical Depression' as: "A psychiatric disorder characterized by an inability to concentrate, insomnia, feelings of extreme sadness, guilt, helplessness and hopelessness, and thoughts of death." A complete loss of appetite might be a symptom or extreme overeating might be a symptom as well.

Depression of obese people is well documented. In studies done by reputable groups, obese people reported that they were treated with less than their due respect even by medical professionals.

Depression is a downward spiral. What begins as just mild depression can descend into the depths of clinical depression. Clinical depression is more prevalent among the obese than it is in the general population.

According to the American Journal of Public Health, Volume 90, Issue 2 251-257 the study, Relationships between obesity and DSM-IV major depressive disorder, suicide ideation, and suicide attempts: results from a general population study done by KM Carpenter, DS Hasin, DB Allison and MS Faith Division of Epidemiology, Joseph L. Mailman School of Public Health, Columbia University, New York, NY, USA, "Relative body weight was associated with major depression, suicide attempts, and suicide ideation, although relationships were different for men and women. Among women, increased BMI was associated with both major depression and suicide ideation. Among men, lower BMI was associated with major depression, suicide attempts, and suicide ideation. There were no racial differences."

**We will discuss BMI (Body Mass Index) in the next chapter but briefly, it is the indicator used by most physicians to determine obesity.

Low self-esteem can affect those who are obese and that low-self esteem can cause them to engage in risky or destructive behaviors. This risky and destructive behavior is more prevalent among obese teenagers with low self-esteem than in other obese populations. Obese teenagers with low self-esteem are more apt to engage in promiscuous sexual activity and alcohol and drug abuse than their average weight peers.

Because obese people are more apt to be discriminated against in housing and employment opportunities, their low self-esteem is exacerbated by society in general. Their self-esteem might have been low when they applied for that job or that apartment and when they are rejected, they blame the rejection on their weighty issue (whether that was the real reason for their rejection or not) and their self-esteem sinks to a new low. This exercise is repeated again and again over the years. It isn't hard to see why obese people are plagued by low self-esteem.

**Obesity Affects Us Socially**

It is sad but all too true fact that society in general views those who are obese as fat, lazy and gluttonous. I wish that weren't true. People should be judged by the fine personal qualities that they have rather on how much they weigh but, unfortunately in the weight conscious world we live in, that simply isn't the case.

Obese individuals are discriminated against in housing markets and in the work place. They are also discriminated against in social situations. Discrimination starts early and lasts a lifetime. The overweight 10-year-old isn't invited to a birthday party. The overweight teenager doesn't have a date for the prom. The overweight young professional isn't included in the after work beer bash. In general, obese people are not included in social events and their invitations didn't get lost in the mail....the invitations were never mailed.

Some obese adults do learn to just accept themselves as they are. They call themselves BBW (Big Beautiful Women) or BHM (Big Handsome Men). Because they do accept themselves they find an acceptable social life....and that is fine if it's true. Others, however, can't accept their obesity with a positive attitude. These obese people find themselves alone and lonely and they aren't happy about it.

**Legalizing Obesity Discrimination**

"No shoes, No shirt, No service" signs might one day be replaced with signs saying "Not Thin don't come in". Already airlines can legally require obese people to purchase two seats on an airplane. Some selected quotes from The Sleaze in the UK are, "The government is adopting a radical new strategy in its war against the scourge of obesity, abandoning attempts to tackle the root causes of the problem directly, it instead aims to stigmatize the overweight. "Look, it's worked with smoking," says Health Minister John Pucker. "By forcing people out on to the street to have a cigarette, the workplace ban on smoking is making it clear to smokers that they are, quite literally, social outcasts." Pucker is keen to see similar measures applied to the grossly overweight, and has welcomed proposals from top doctors to deny fertility treatment to the obese."

"First England and then the rest of the world", as the old saying goes, may apply to legalizing obesity discrimination.

Conclusion: Obesity affects adults and children physically, mentally, emotionally and socially. Obesity discrimination is becoming legal in more and more circumstances.

When we set out to change our weight we are in reality changing much more than our weight. We are taking the first steps toward a drastic life style change. This is especially true for those who have more than a few pounds to lose. A person who loses thirty, forty, fifty or more pounds will not be the same person they were before they lost the weight. They will not react to the world around them the same and the world around them will not react to them the same. They will not want to participate in the same activities that they participated in when they were heavy. They won't even laugh at the same jokes.

It is true, as well, that successfully losing weight requires a lot of outside support. We all look to our family and friends for support in many aspects of our lives but losing weight is one endeavor that really does require the support of others who are traveling or have traveled the same path. Although our family and friends may well want to give us their full support while we lose those many unwanted pounds, they aren't the ones who can understand or appreciate the day to day (sometimes minute to minute) struggles and temptations that we face.

When you combine the facts of life style change with the need for support, the obvious solution of the combined needs is a weight loss support group.

A weight loss support group need not be one of the well-known ones that we will be discussing here. A weight loss support group can be a loosely knit group of people who join together in a joint effort to lose weight and support one another in the process. Many such groups are formed just among groups of friends or among groups of co-workers everyday and many are very successful.

Weight loss support groups offer the opportunity for those wanting and needing to lose weight to form new friendships, to learn about food and exercise from one another, to give and get support, and one more important thing....they provide an opportunity to win.

Friendships are naturally formed between people who have common goals. Solid bonds can be formed between people who under other circumstances would never become allies when they are faced with a common enemy....in this instance over weight....the battle of the bulge.....food temptations. These things become the common enemy of a weight loss group and friendships are the natural product of fighting a common enemy.

Learning about food and how it affects weight is one of the main goals of most weight loss support groups. Important and helpful information is presented at meetings of weight loss support groups on many topics that affect the loss of weight as well as the problem of keeping on keeping on in the face of adversity. Programs are presented on such varied topics as 'The Importance of Drinking Water' to 'How to Spot a Diet Sabotage in the Making'. Most weight loss support groups teach the importance of keeping food diaries. They give instruction about counting calories, fat grams and carb grams, as well. Usually programs are presented by different members of the group from week to week and, as we all know, you learn more by teaching than you ever learn by being taught.

Exercise is not only encouraged in weight loss support groups, many groups provide for group exercise or group walking sessions. Exercise not only makes you sweat it is usually downright boring....and misery loves company. It's a lot easier to put on those walking shoes and go for that walk if your friends are waiting for you and will be walking with you than it is to just get out of your comfy easy chair and go alone.

Support given and received from the members of a weight loss support group is an invaluable asset in the pursuit of weight loss. Everyone who has ever had to lose more than a few pounds knows all about the dreaded 'plateau' of weight loss. You will go along for a few weeks and lose one or two pounds at a steady clip and then all of a sudden and for no apparent reason, you lose not one ounce even though you have done the same thing as you have done in weeks past. A word of encouragement can help you stick with your plan when it doesn't look like it is working. Having a friend to call when that piece of cake in the fridge is calling to you to help you resist temptation is priceless.

The opportunity to win a challenge or a competition is another thing that weight loss support groups provide. When most people are faced with a competition they immediately want to win that competition. It's just human nature. Our own success is always measured against the success of others who are trying to gain the same goals that we are. We start really young learning all about competition through sibling rivalry and we never stop needing to win throughout our lives. Winning equals success. That's why we play games. We don't play for fun...we play to WIN!

It has been proven time and time again that those who face the need to make big behavioral changes in their lives are much more likely to make those changes if they have the support of a group of people who need to make the same changes. Natural weight loss means that behaviors need to be changed. You have to learn to think like a thin person and sea food the way that thin people do. A support group can help you make those changes.

There are many organized support groups to choose from. I am not advocating any particular group here. You many well want to visit different groups and see where you feel the most comfortable and which one you think will help you the very most. We will discuss three prominent programs here (Weight Watchers, Tops, and Overeaters Anonymous) but be aware that there are others.

**Obesity Research**

We are all waiting with bated breath for the scientific community to finally come up with the reason for obesity and a magic pill that will just FIX it. There are naturally thin people that walk this planet. Why doesn't somebody just put them under a microscope and figure out why THEY can eat everything but the stove and still be thin and the rest of us can't and then find the way to make all of us like that?

Actually research into the reasons for obesity and possible cures for it are going on all the time. If you really want to become part of an obesity research project, you can find which ones are looking for test subjects by going to Google and typing in "obesity research clinical trials" or going to the American Obesity Association website's research page.

You will find that most of the research projects and studies being done are related to behavioral changes. That is because most obesity is caused by over eating or under exercising or both.

There are other studies and research projects in progress now or planned for the future that focus on physical reasons for obesity as opposed to behavioral causes and there are those that really looking for that magic pill we all dream of.

Several such studies that are now recruiting test subjects are:

• The Role of the Orexin System in Body Weight

• Chronic Sleep Deprivation as a Risk Factor for Metabolic Syndrome and Obesity

• Body Heat Content and Dissipation in Obese and Normal Weight Adults

• Peripheral Thyroid Hormone Conversion and Glucose and Energy Metabolism

• Eating Behavior in Children

• Effects of Metformin on Energy Intake, Energy Expenditure, and Body Weight in Overweight Children with Insulin Resistance

The above list is a partial one. There are always research projects and studies being conducted at medical facilities and research departments at colleges around the country. Someday maybe somebody will come up with a magic fix for the problem of obesity but I won't be holding my breath on that one.

All research proves that reduced intake of calories and increased expenditure of calories equal weight loss and that accomplishing those two things naturally is the best and safest way to lose weight.

**Tips and Tools for Natural Weight Loss**

If you have read what has been written in the book so far, there shouldn't be much doubt in your mind that losing those excess pounds is the wisest course of action for you and that losing that weight naturally is by far the safest way to go.

Here are some tips and tools to help you lose those unwanted pounds and do it the natural way. Let's start with tools:

1. A Pair of Scales: It is imperative that you have a method to chart your weight loss. You need a starting weight and then you need to see progress to help you maintain your resolve to continue. You can purchase a pair of bathroom scales for a small amount of money at your nearest discount store. Of course, you can pay any amount that you choose to pay for a pair of scales. You can even get them that talk to you but it really isn't necessary to have an absolute accurate weight. What matters is that you can measure weight LOSS. Even if the scales weigh a little heavy or a little light, it doesn't matter much. They can still tell you if you are gaining or losing weight.

2. A Tape Measure: On the morning that you begin your quest for weight loss and finding a way to eat healthier, take your body measurements. Measure your chest, waist and hips, of course, but you also need to measure your thighs, calves and upper and lower arms. You can most likely accomplish this yourself in the privacy of your own bathroom but you need to write those measurements down so that you can see the reductions in the measurements as you progress. Many times you will not see a weight loss on the scales but can measure a loss of inches with a tape measure.

3. A Set of Measuring Cups: The number of calories/fat/carbohydrates in food is determined by the quantity...not just by the name of the food. In order to effectively measure the number of calories/fat/carbohydrates in the food you consume, you are going to have to measure your portions. **Note: all food is measured loosely not packed. A half cup of rice, for example, is first fluffed with a fork and then spooned into a measuring cup and leveled with the back of a knife.

4. A Food Scale: You can purchase a simple food scale at your nearest discount store for just a few dollars or you can buy one that will not only weigh the food but calculate the calories in it.

This is another one of those items that you can spend as much as you want to on. You can even find them that can be mounted on a wall. Nothing elaborate is really needed if you passed third grade math, however. If you know how many calories are in an ounce of cooked beef, you can easily multiply by 4 if there are four ounces in what you are planning on eating.

These are the only four tools that you will ever need to successfully lose weight and then keep from gaining it back. Even if you are going to use a diet plan that provides prepackaged meals to lose weight, you will eventually need to be able to weigh and measure foods that you prepare at home. A pair of scales and a tape measure is needed no matter what kind of diet you are going to use.

**Tips for Natural Weight Loss Success**

1. Make a Plan: Those who fail to plan, plan to fail...that is an old saying but it is an accurate one. Unless you are following a diet plan that provides prepackaged food, you will need to sit down each evening after dinner and plan what you will be 'allowed' to eat the following day. This plan will help to keep you from overeating or eating things that are not on your list for the day.

2. Keep a food diary: Calories are so sneaky. They are everywhere even in the most innocent looking food. The rule you need to follow to keep your food diary is that before you put anything into your mouth you write it down. Keep your food diary handy...you don't want to have to look for it. A food diary can tell you many things. You can find the hidden calories or you can find the ones that you can eliminate painlessly if your food diary is complete and accurate.

3. Keep a Journal: This can be kept in the same notebook that you use for your food diary or it can be separate. I have found that each relates to the other but does it your way...just do it. Start your diet journal by writing down the date and your feelings about yourself. Use your journal to record the foods that you eat, when you eat them and why you eat them. This journal can be a key that will help you unlock your inner feelings that cause you to overeat and help you to overcome temptations when they arise...and they WILL arise. Write something in your journal everyday whether you think it relates to your diet or not....EVERYTHING relates to your diet. A call from a friend, a work related problem or a spat with your sister all affect how you feel about yourself and how you feel about yourself affects every aspect of your life including your diet.

4. Set Goals: Goals come in two varieties. There are long term goals and there are short term goals. Long term goals are realized by achieving short term goals. For example: Let's say you want to lose 40 pounds. Losing 40 pounds is a long term goal. It isn't going to happen next week. A short term goal is to lose 1 pound. That is a doable short term goal. So make two lists....one for long term goals and don't limit this list to just weight loss....think about what you would like to accomplish in your life.

You might want to learn a foreign language or travel abroad or learn to knit. It doesn't matter what your long term goals are as long as they are things that will make you fell happier. The second list will have to be made every week. This short term list are the baby steps that you need to take in order to reach your long term goals. Look at your long term list and make your short term list. For example: You might put 'lose 1 pound' on your short term list. You might also put, 'check out French Lesson Tapes from library' or 'Get travel brochure. The way that long term goals are met are by meeting short terms goals often enough to get there. It's the way that all great things are accomplished by human beings. Only God can create instant miracles.

5. Make an Exercise Plan: You can only reduce your intake of calories just so far. You have to eat so a plan to eat less AND exercise more is the better way to plan to lose weight. Exercise can't be done only when the mood strikes you....it won't strike. You need to set aside a time (or more than one time) each day to exercise in whatever way you choose. Remember when you were a kid? You exercised then...you just called it 'play' and it was what you did that was fun. The same is true now that you are all grown up. Your exercise shouldn't be a burden but rather something that you can enjoy and challenge yourself with. Choose an exercise that will give you satisfaction and even pleasure. If you choose walking as an exercise then find a walking partner that you love to be with and one that can make you laugh.

6. Reward Yourself: Remember those goals we talked about? When you reach a goal...a short term one even....give yourself a pat on the back. It might sound silly but buy yourself some stick on gold stars and put one on your journal page when you lose a pound or when you exercise every day. Write in big bold letters YEA! GOOD FOR ME! Reward yourself even more for each 5 pounds of weight lose. Buy yourself a new pair of earrings or a new scarf or a wallet. Have you nails done....whatever makes you feel good about yourself is a reward....just NOT FOOD. Never ever use food as a reward. For a 10 pound weight loss make the reward even bigger and better.

7. Get Support: Losing weight is a hard and sometimes lonely thing. When we are in the midst of doing battle with ourselves and effecting life altering changes we need support. We can't do it all by ourselves. Join one of the Weight loss support groups that we discussed back in Chapter VI....either one in the brick and mortar

world or one that is as close as the computer that you are reading this book on.

8. Forgive Yourself: We all fail sometimes. One little failure, however, is not reason enough to quip altogether. So you had a weak moment and ate something that you shouldn't have or you got lazy and skipped an exercise appointment with yourself....just forgive yourself, promise you that you will do better and stay with your weight loss program. The rewards for success are worth every bit of the effort.

# About the Author

Timothy Campbell is a health buff and a well-known fitness instructor. His over ten years of experience made him one of the best instructors in the country. Timothy Campbell wants to continue inspiring and helping others, that's why he wrote this book to reach out to others on a global scale.

Timothy is married to Alexa who is a holistic instructor and they live in Oregon.

www.ingramcontent.com/pod-product-compliance
Lightning Source LLC
Chambersburg PA
CBHW070028260726

48658CB00002B/541